The UMAP Expository Monograph Series

UMAP Monographs bring the undergraduate student new mathematics and fresh applications of mathematics with no delay between the development of an idea and its implementation in the undergraduate curriculum.

Spatial Models of Election Competition
Steven J. Brams, *New York University*

Elements of the Theory of Generalized Inverses for Matrices
Randall E. Cline, *University of Tennessee*

Introduction to Population Modeling
James C. Frauenthal, *SUNY at Stony Brook*

Smallpox: When Should Routine Vaccination be Discontinued?
James C. Frauenthal, *SUNY at Stony Brook*

Conditional Independence in Applied Probability
Paul E. Pfeiffer, *Rice University*

Topics in the Theory of Voting
Philip D. Straffin, Jr., *Beloit College*

Man in Competition with the Spruce Budworm:
An Application of Differential Equations
Philip M. Tuchinsky, *Ford Motor Company's Research and Engineering Center*

James C. Frauenthal

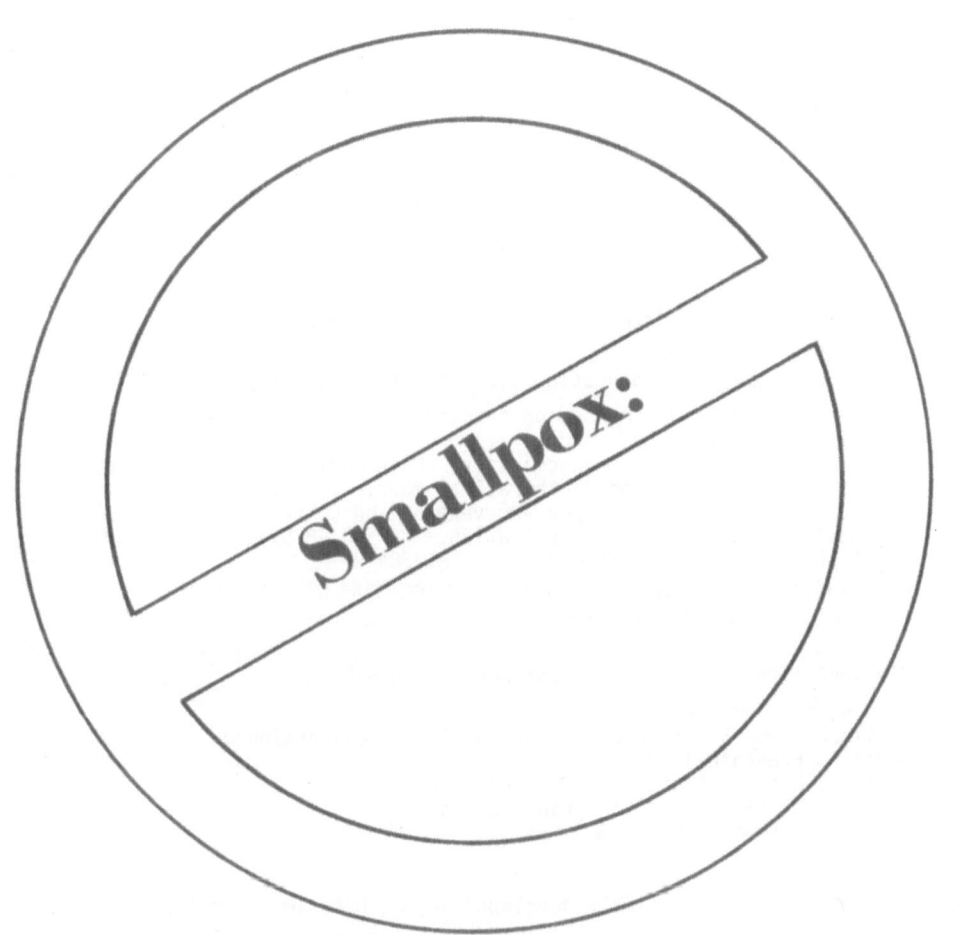

When Should Routine
Vaccination Be Discontinued?

BIRKHÄUSER

BOSTON • BASEL • STUTTGART

Author:

James C. Frauenthal
Applied Mathematics and Statistics
State University of New York
Stony Brook, New York 11794

Library of Congress Cataloging in Publication Data

Frauenthal, J.C., 1944-
  Smallpox, when should routine vaccination be discontinued?

  (The UMAP expository monograph series)
  Bibliography: p.
  1. Smallpox--Preventive inoculation-- Mathematical Models.
2. Smallpox--Transmission--Mathematical models. I. Title.
II. Series. (DNLM: 1. Smallpox--Prevention and Control.
2. Models, Structural. 3. Vaccination. WC 588 F845s)
RA644.S6F7   614.5'21'0724   81-38439
ISBN-13: 978-0-8176-3042-3   e-ISBN-13: 978-1-4684-6719-2   AACR2
DOI: 10.1007/978-1-4684-6719-2

CIP-Kurztitelaufnahme der Deutschen Bibliothek

Frauenthal, James C.:
Smallpox: When Should Routine Vaccination Be Discontinued?
James C. Frauenthal.-
Boston ; Basel ; Stuttgart : Birkhaeuser, 1981
  (The UMAP Expository Monograph Series)
  ISBN-13: 978-0-8176-3042-3   .

This material was initially developed in the Department of Applied
Mathematics and Statistics at State University of New York,
Stony Brook (NSF Grant No. SED76-05433), and has continued development
under UMAP with the partial support of National Science Foundation
Grant No. SED80-07731. Recommendations expressed are those of the
author and do not necessarily reflect the views of the NSF or the
copyright holder.

Table of Contents

Eradication of Smallpox
To Be Announced Today

Special to The New York Times

UNITED NATIONS, N.Y., May 7 — Smallpox, one of the deadliest and oldest viral diseases of humans, has been eradicated from the earth, World Health Organization officials said today in a news conference broadcast here from Geneva.

The death of smallpox, which had been reported in stages over the last two years, marks the first time in history that the natural transmission of a disease has been completely stopped. Public health leaders have hailed the accomplishment as a milestone in medicine.

The official declaration of the eradication of smallpox will be made in ceremonies tomorrow at the World Health Assembly, now being held in Geneva.

The health organization began the intensified smallpox eradication program in 1967. In that year, smallpox was reported in 42 countries and killed two million people. It also scarred and blinded another eight million people.

An immediate effect of the eradication program has been to make smallpox vaccinations needless, thereby eliminating the risks from that centuries-old procedure. Also, no person will need to have evidence of a smallpox vaccination for travel to any country at any time.

The Last Case Of Smallpox: An Old Story, Told Again

BY HAROLD M. SCHMECK JR.

The driver of the Land Rover had two children with smallpox in the back seat. He needed directions to the isolation camp near Merka, Somalia.

The young man who gave him directions, spending less than 10 minutes in the vehicle with the driver and two patients, was a cook in the hospital at Merka, a town of about 20,000 near the southern extremity of the Horn of Africa.

That brief chance encounter last October may have made the cook, 23-year-old Ali Maaow Maalin, the last human being to become a victim of smallpox.

After helping the driver find the smallpox eradication team leader in Merka, the cook went back to work at the hospital and let the matter slip from his mind.

Two weeks later he developed a fever and was sent home to rest. Two days after that, still feverish, he was back in the hospital as a patient. His illness was first diagnosed as malaria, then as chicken pox.

During all that time, both at home and in the hospital, he had visitors. No one recalled that he had been exposed to two active cases of smallpox. No one checked his vaccination record.

But soon it became all too obvious that he had smallpox and was a living, contagious threat to one of the world's great public health accomplishments.

For more than 10 years, doctors and other public health workers throughout the world had been fighting humanity's first successful war of annihilation against an infectious disease. Under the leadership of the World Health Organization the global total of smallpox cases was reduced from 2½ million in 1976 to almost zero by the fall of 1977.

The health organization certified the eradication of smallpox from the Americas in 1973, Indonesia in 1974, 15 West African countries as well as Pakistan and Afghanistan in 1976, and the rest of Asia and Central Africa last year. Certification means that there had been no cases during the two previous years and that the chain of infection had presumably been broken. The last nonimported cases in the United States were in 1949.

By last fall only the Horn of Africa seemed to remain as a last stronghold of a contagious scourge that maimed and killed millions of human beings for at least 3,000 years.

But then came the case of the hospital cook in Merka. From the point of view of containing the disease, the young man was about as bad a case as could be imagined. He worked in a hospital in a city that had continual traffic with a much bigger city — Mogadishu. The delay in identifying the cause of his illness offered plenty of chance for further spread.

The smallpox eradication team in Merka had to track down every single one of his contacts.

Dr. Jason S. Weisfeld of the United States' Center for Disease Control in Atlanta was part of that effort and dealt with that case. He said Ali Maaow Maalin had had more than 160 contacts during the period in which he might have been infectious and before the nature of his disease was recognized. Each one was tracked down. It turned out that most of them had been vaccinated and therefore posed no threat of further spread, but 33 had had face-to-face exposure and no previous vaccination.

Meanwhile, the young cook recovered and went back to work. Public health workers burned his mattress, sheets and personal articles from the room where he had spent the period of his illness.

Each week for the first three weeks a search for new smallpox cases was made in every place he and his potentially infectious contacts might have visited. Then there was a search every two weeks, Dr. Weisfeld said, and, since November, every month.

No new case has been found. The hospital employee's illness is officially dated Oct. 26, 1977. Since then no case of smallpox has been discovered anywhere in the world. Never before in history has there been a period of six months with no reported smallpox.

But is the long terrible story of smallpox really ended?

Specialists in this dread disease are by no means willing to claim final victory yet. War between Ethiopia and Somalia in the Horn of Africa has seriously hampered the surveillance effort. Furthermore, the area of concern is a region of nomads and obscure villages where mild cases of smallpox might persist without the knowledge of the public health teams that try to comb the area.

The Center for Disease Control in Atlanta, at present the world's center for laboratory diagnosis of smallpox, continues to get specimens from Africa, each representing another suspicious illness.

One such shipment was brought back a week ago by Dr. Stanley D. Foster of the center, who had been in Somalia working on the smallpox surveillance effort. These cases seemed highly suspicious, but laboratory tests have ruled them out. They were not smallpox.

Still, the doubts remain, largely because of the war. Smallpox and war have often been linked in the past. One of the tragic ironies of this last fight against that ancient enemy of mankind, smallpox, is that the victory may be compromised, and is at least obscured, by that other ancient plague, war.

Harold M. Schmeck Jr. writes on science for The New York Times.

Preface

The material discussed in this monograph should be
accessible to upper level undergraduates in the mathematical sciences. Formal prerequisites include a solid introduction to calculus and one semester of probability.
Although differential equations are employed, these are all
linear, constant coefficient, ordinary differential equations which are solved either by separation of variables or
by introduction of an integrating factor. These techniques
can be taught in a few minutes to students who have studied
calculus. The models developed to describe an epidemic
outbreak of smallpox are standard stochastic processes
(birth-death, random walk and branching processes). While
it would be helpful for students to have seen these prior
to their introduction in this monograph, it is certainly
not necessary. The stochastic processes are developed from
first principles and then solved using elementary techniques. Since all that turns out to be necessary are expected values of random variables, the differential-difference equation descriptions of the stochastic processes are
reduced to ordinary differential equations before being
solved.

Students who have studied stochastic processes are
generally pleased to learn that different formulations are
possible for the same set of conditions. The choice of
which formulation to employ depends upon what one wishes to
calculate. Specifically, in Section 6 a birth-death process is replaced by a random walk and in Section 7 a problem is formulated both as a multi-birth-death process and
as a branching process.

I would like to take this opportunity to express my thanks to Norman T.J. Bailey, Chief of the Health Statistical Methodology Section of the World Health Organization, Geneva who called my attention to the very timely and interesting set of mathematical models contained in this monograph. I would also like to thank Stavros Busenberg of the Department of Mathematics at Harvey Mudd College in Claremont, California who read through the manuscripts for this monograph and made numerous useful suggestions. Finally, I would like to thank the National Science Foundation whose support under Grant SED76-05433 greatly aided in the production of this monograph.

Stony Brook, N.Y.   James C. Frauenthal
January, 1981

Introduction

One of the most remarkable accomplishments in the history of preventive medicine has recently taken place. A global campaign by the World Health Organization appears to have successfully eradicated smallpox, one of the most terrible of human diseases, from the earth. Since 1977, there has not been a single case of normally transmitted smallpox reported anywhere in the world (though there were two cases, one fatal, following a laboratory accident in Britain in 1978). If smallpox has indeed been eliminated, it will be the first time in the history of mankind that such a feat has been achieved.

Interestingly, there is still no known cure for smallpox. Even with modern medical procedures, roughly 10% of the people who contract the disease die from it, and those who survive are usually badly scarred. The World Health Organization program to eradicate smallpox made use of a vaccine which provides immunity to the disease for several years. By any reasonable medical standard, this vaccine is safe, effective, inexpensive, and nearly painless to receive. Yet in 1971, with smallpox still endemic in more than a dozen countries, the United States suspended routine vaccination of children about to enroll in school. Why was this decision made?

A closer look at the epidemiological record provides some insight. The last case of smallpox transmitted in the United States occurred in 1949. Nearly twenty years later, in 1968 (a year for which detailed records are available -- see Lane, et. al., 1969) a total of about 14,168,000 individuals were vaccinated against smallpox. Although the average cost and risk to each individual was very small,

the high number of vaccinations caused the total estimated
cost of vaccine production, record keeping, doctors' ser-
vices, ..., to amount to $150,000,000. In addition, 572
persons developed complications serious enough to be reported to public health authorities, and 9 individuals died
from the vaccine.

If in retrospect the amount of money spent on, and the
number of complications and fatalities resulting from,
needless vaccination in the United States since 1949 (and
in the world since 1977) seems absurd, it may quite logi-
cally be attributed to fear. After all, in 1967, the year
before the vaccination statistics quoted in the last para-
graph, smallpox had killed two million people and scarred
or blinded eight million more over the globe, and the World
Health Organization's campaign had just begun.

The problem to be addressed is the following: when
does the risk of a serious but rare disease for which there
is a prevention but no cure become sufficiently small that
it is better not to use preventive measures, even if prevention is extremely safe? A number of diseases satisfy
the general requirements: poliomyelitis, measles, influenza, and until its very recent eradication, smallpox.

Since the details of the mathematical models which aid
in making the decision about whether to take preventive
measures are highly disease- and vaccine-specific, it is
necessary to select a disease in advance and study its
characteristics. The remainder of this monograph will
concentrate on smallpox. This choice was made for several
reasons. Smallpox has been one of the worst of human
scourges for millennia, and has only recently been eradicated. The question of when to stop vaccinating against
smallpox has occupied public health officials for many
years. Smallpox is also interesting because it has been
discussed at length in the popular press during the eradication campaign. More about the history of smallpox will
be found in Section 2, (The History of Smallpox
Vaccination). Another reason for choosing smallpox is that
it has several mathematically suitable epidemiological features. These features, some of which made smallpox eradication possible, are discussed in Section 3 (The
Epidemiology of Smallpox).

It is worth reiterating that the choice of smallpox as
the disease to model affects the details of this monograph,
but not the general idea that mathematical models can be
employed in epidemiological decision-making.

1 The History of Smallpox Vaccination

It has apparently been understood since ancient times
that smallpox produces its own natural immunity: anyone who
survives a case of the disease is immune to subsequent infection. A technique called variolation was used long ago
in India and China to produce artificial resistance to
smallpox. This technique consisted of innoculating a susceptible individual with variola virus taken from a smallpox pustule on an active case. If successful, the result
of variolation was a very mild case which left the innoculated individual immune. The case of smallpox was usually
mild because the ordinary transmission route of the disease
through the atmosphere and into the respiratory system of
the victim was short-circuited by the direct application of
the virus to the skin. If variolation was unsuccessful,
the innoculated individual might contract a severe, disfig-
uring case of smallpox and even die, or might be left with
no added immunity from the innoculation. At best, variolation was a risky way to prevent smallpox, but it was the
only way.

The practice of variolation was brought to Europe ear-
ly in the eighteenth century. The introduction of the
technique makes for an interesting story of unlikely cir-
cumstances profoundly affecting history. It seems that a
wealthy and very beautiful English woman named Mary
Pierrepont eloped (against her father's wishes) with Edward
Mortley Montagu, grandson of the first Earl of Sandwich.
In 1715, Edward was elected to Parliament and Mary contracted smallpox, which left her sadly scarred. The next
year Edward was appointed Ambassador to the Turkish court.
While in Constantinople, Lady Mary learned of the Turkish

practice of variolation; she was sufficiently impressed to risk having her own children variolated. When she returned to London in 1718, she used her knowledge and position to campaign vigorously for variolation. Perhaps more than anyone else, Lady Mary was responsible for bringing variolation to England and subsequently to Europe and the United States. (For a truly fascinating account of variolation, see Langer, 1976).

It is interesting to note that the first documented use of mathematics in epidemiology was concerned with evaluating the effectiveness of variolation. The famous Swiss scientist Daniel Bernoulli presented the results of a mathematical model for smallpox innoculation to the Academie Royale des Sciences in Paris in April of 1760. (The interested reader can find an English translation of this paper in Bradley, 1971, and an account of a resulting controversy with Jean LeRonde d'Alembert in Bailey, 1975. Since the Bernoulli model is not especially pertinent to the present problem, it will not be discussed further here, though Exercise 1 is designed to guide the reader through Bernoulli's modelling process and some of its results.)

Toward the end of the eighteenth century, Edward Jenner, a country physician in England, observed that women who worked around cows did not often contract smallpox. He conjectured that the reason was that they caught a mild case of cowpox, the bovine form of smallpox. Since the cowpox infections were so mild as to yield no symptoms other than smallpox immunity, Jenner developed an immunization procedure vastly superior to classic variolation.[1] This method, which is still used with only minor changes, consisted of variolation with cowpox virus; the technique came to be called vaccination, and was so effective that Jenner predicted it would lead to the eventual annihilation of smallpox. During the first 150 years after its introduction, widespread vaccination became the primary weapon in the battle against smallpox. In the United States, for example, smallpox was virtually eliminated by requiring all children to be vaccinated before enrolling in school. By the late 1930's only occasional outbreaks still occurred; since 1949, not a single case has been contracted in the United States.

The European experience with smallpox has been only slightly less favorable. The next two examples are typical of the several dozen small epidemics that have occurred in parts of Europe over the past 25 years. The January 1970 outbreak in Meschede, West Germany, described in detail in the next section, resulted in 20 cases and 4 deaths. A rather more serious epidemic, which began in England in the winter of 1961-62, caused 24 deaths and resulted in the expenditure of nearly $4,000,000 for preventive vaccination and hospital care.

The worldwide incidence of smallpox remained a topic of major concern as recently as twenty years ago. In 1958, the World Health Organization began its smallpox eradication program. Recognizing the impossibility of vaccinating every human being in the world, they concentrated their efforts on locating and isolating smallpox cases, and then tracing all possible infective contacts for prompt vaccination and possible quarantine (later in the campaign, they addressed the problem of unreported cases by offering a bounty of $1,000 for discovery of a smallpox case). By 1966, only 43 nations reported any incidence of smallpox, and the disease was considered endemic (continuously occurring) only in 28 of them. By 1970, the numbers had declined to 21 and 14 nations respectively. And on May 7, 1980, World Health Organization officials held a news conference in Geneva in which they announced the end of smallpox on earth. (More about the eradication campaign can be found in articles by Breman and Arita, 1980, Henderson 1976, and Stockton, 1979; the latter also discusses the currently remaining problem of security in smallpox research laboratories stocking the virus.)

2 The Epidemiology of Smallpox

Smallpox is caused by a virus which is transmitted only between humans. There is no known reservoir for the disease among other species of animals.[2] Consequently, if an isolated region is smallpox free, the only way for the disease to occur is by importation. Specifically, someone susceptible to smallpox must contract it in a region where the disease is found and then travel to the smallpox free region. Unfortunately, as with most viral diseases, there is a period of time between initial infection and the appearance of externally observable symptoms. As a result, an infected individual can innocently transmit the disease to susceptible individuals before the disease is identified.

For smallpox, the contagious but asymptomatic period lasts about five days on average. So with jet travel, an infected individual can reach any point in the world before becoming aware of the disease. An added recent difficulty results from the rareness of smallpox; when a case does begin to manifest itself, local health officials may be slow to make proper identification and thus slow to take proper precautions.

Once the disease is identified, containing the epidemic is ordinarily not too difficult, even though smallpox is highly contagious. There are a number of reasons for this. Modern rapid communication permits easy notification of public health authorities, and also facilitates tracing all contacts that the infected individual may have made. In addition, since most hospital workers and medical personnel maintain their immunity through regular vaccination, the infective can be effectively isolated from susceptible individuals. As secondary cases (those transmitted by the initial infective) appear, they can be readily identified and isolated. It is therefore safe to assume that any smallpox epidemic which might get started in a highly developed nation would be limited to a few hundred cases at most. The risk of a "pandemic" simply no longer exists. This assertion is supported by evidence from the last minor smallpox epidemics in Europe.

To help illustrate the dynamics of the disease, let us consider the smallpox epidemic in Meschede, West Germany, in 1970. (For a highly detailed account, see Brown, 1971). The epidemic was begun by a 20 year old West German male who had wandered and apparently slept in the streets of Karachi, Pakistan for 3 days in late December, 1969. He returned to his home in Meschede on 31 December 1969, ill with hepatitis. In his possession was a valid smallpox vaccination certificate; apparently the vaccination had not been successful. On January 10 he developed fever and was admitted to a private room in the infectious isolation ward of Meschede Hospital, with his condition diagnosed as typhoid fever. On 14 January a rash developed, and smallpox was confirmed on 16 January. The patient was transferred to a special isolation hospital in another city.

After the diagnosis of smallpox, all people known to have had contact with the initial infective were vaccinated immediately. In addition, during the next few days, all patients and workers in the Meschede hospital were vaccinated. The wing of the hospital that contained the isolation ward was quarantined, with no one allowed in or out except for transfer to other isolation facilities after signs of smallpox appeared.

Between 22 and 31 January, 17 additional cases of smallpox developed. Interestingly, although all of these people had been in the wing of the Meschede Hospital where the primary case occurred, none had had any direct contact with the initial infective. Two further cases appeared between 13 and 16 February in hospital roommates of individuals in the earlier outbreak. Fortunately, no cases occurred due to contacts with the initial infective prior to his admission to the hospital.

Table 1 shows the sequence of cases in the Meschede Hospital epidemic, along with relevant facts concerning age and sex of the victim, dates of onset of disease, prior vaccination record and outcome. Note that three of the four deaths that ultimately resulted were among elderly people who were hospital patients at the time they contracted smallpox. The fourth victim who died was a young nurse who had no record of vaccination before 16 January.

TABLE 1*

Cases of Smallpox – Meschede Hospital, 1970

Case No.	Age	Sex	Onset		Outcome	Past Vaccination		Comment
			Fever	Rash		Vacc. scar	Most recent vacc. (year)	
1	20	M	10 Jan.	14 Jan.		No	1969	Index patient-ground floor
2	5	F	23 Jan.	25 Jan.		No	--	Patient-ground floor
3	17	F	22 Jan.	25 Jan.	Death	No	--	Nurse-third floor
4	21	F	25 Jan.	28 Jan.		No	--	Nurse-second floor
5	57	M	22 Jan.	26 Jan.		Yes	1968	Patient-third floor
6	50	F	25 Jan.	29 Jan.		Yes	1932	Patient-ground floor
7	56	M	26 Jan.	29 Jan.		Yes	1942	Patient-second floor
8	42	M	24 Jan.	26 Jan.		Yes	1946	Visitor on 13 Jan.
9	79	M	27 Jan.	29 Jan.	Death	Yes	1903(?)	Patient-second floor
10	89	M	28 Jan.	30 Jan.		Yes	--	Patient-third floor
11	90	M	28 Jan.	30 Jan.		Yes	1892(?)	Patient-second floor
12	59	M	28 Jan.	31 Jan.		Yes	1930	Patient-third floor
13	73	M	31 Jan.	1 Feb.		Yes	1909	Patient-third floor
14	59	F	29 Jan.	2 Feb.		Yes	1930	Nurse-third floor
15	65	F	31 Jan.	2 Feb.		Yes	1917	Patient-third floor
16	69	F	31 Jan.	2 Feb.		Yes	1902	Patient-ground floor
17	60	M	31 Jan.	4 Feb.	Death	Yes	1917	Patient-second floor
18	21	M	22 Jan.	None		Yes	1961	Patient-second floor
19	74	M	13 Feb.	15 Feb.		Yes	1907(?)	Patient-contact:case 17
20	81	F	16 Feb.	17 Feb.	Death	Yes	1901(?)	Patient-contact:case 15

*Reproduced from Gelfand and Posch, in Brown, 1971.

The Meschede epidemic is probably typical of what
would happen if smallpox were imported to the United
States. Obviously, the severity of the outbreak would depend on a variety of factors, including the level of susceptibility in the exposed population and the frequency of
contacts by the infectives prior to disease identification.

The question that will be addressed by mathematical
analysis is whether the level of susceptibility in a
population should be permitted to rise, perhaps even to its
natural unprotected level, as the likelihood of a serious
disease diminishes due to reduced worldwide incidence. In
the next section, the structure of a mathematical model is
formulated. This model was originally presented in a paper
written by Niels Becker (1972).

3 The Mathematical Model
Introduction

It is convenient to visualize the outbreak of a local-
ized smallpox epidemic as taking place in three stages. In
the first stage the region to be considered is disease-
free, and the population is maintained at a predetermined
level of susceptibility by an ongoing vaccination program.
Typically this stage lasts for several years. In Section 5
(the Pre-Epidemic Model) we will develop an expression for
the expected number $E\{m\}$ of deaths caused by smallpox vaccinations prior to the disease importation.

The second stage begins with the arrival of a smallpox
infected person. Since present day travel times are quite
short when compared with the incubation times for smallpox,
the infected person initially shows no external symptoms of
the disease. Consequently, the infected individual acci-
dentally comes in contact with susceptible individuals,
spreading the disease. This phase of the epidemic may last
from a few days to perhaps two weeks, and ends when the
first case of smallpox is clearly identified and isolated.
In Section 6 (The Epidemic Initiation Model) we develop an
expression for $E\{Y\}$, the expected number of unidentified
cases of smallpox in the population at the time the first
case is identified.

The third stage of the epidemic corresponds to the
tracing of all of the contacts from the identified case.
Clearly, once public health and medical authorities are
alert to the risk of further cases of the disease, great
care is taken to isolate all possible infectives. With
modern communications and medical care, all infected individuals are typically identified and isolated in just a few
weeks. At this point, the small epidemic will run its

course, and the process will be back at the beginning, waiting for another importation of the disease. In Section 7 (The Epidemic Subsidence Model) we construct a model to estimate the expected number of cases of smallpox caused by the epidemic outbreak.

The three stages of an epidemic are described by separate mathematical models. Once the three models are analyzed, the solutions must be combined so that the total impact of the level of vaccination can be assessed. To combine the solutions, however, it is necessary to calculate a single quantity for each stage of the epidemic. Two alternative choices seem reasonable: total cost in money (dollars), or total cost in human lives. Although either alternative could be justified, it is somewhat easier to deal directly with minimizing the loss of life. This choice is also appealing in that it is closely related to the primary purpose of preventive medicine. In Section 8 (The Optimal Vaccination Policy) we determine an expression for the total number of deaths due to both vaccination and a smallpox epidemic. This expression is then used to find the vaccination rate that minimizes the expected total number of deaths. In Section 9 (Calibrating the Model) the necessary vaccination and disease parameters are estimated for the United States, and conclusions are drawn about optimal vaccination rates given those parameters.

Before undertaking the formulation and solution of these mathematical models, it seems worthwhile to make one additional generalization about them that will describe the epidemic outbreak. Quite simply, when the disease is carried by an unidentified infective, we assume that just two things can happen. Either the infective can spread the disease to susceptible individuals, or the infective can be removed from circulation (because smallpox symptoms appear or because cautious public health authorities quarantine suspected infectives even before the appearance of symptoms). Three completely different mathematical models will be used to describe these simple alternatives.

The choice of models depends on our viewpoint and affects what we are able to determine. The first epidemic model that will be described (in Section 6) is called a birth-death stochastic process. In the context of an epidemic, the name is a bit confusing: a "birth" is a contact which leads to one additional case of the disease; a "death" is the identification and subsequent isolation of one case of the disease. For this type of model, continuous clock time is the independent variable, the current number of unidentified infectives is the dependent random variable, and the solution to the model is the corresponding family of probability density functions (for all values

of the random variable as functions of time). It will turn
out that this formulation is not sufficient to determine
the desired results for this phase of the epidemic, and an
alternative model will be proposed to describe exactly the
same physical situation.

This second model will be called a random walk. A
random walk is another standard stochastic model.
Typically one visualizes a drunkard who staggers forward
and backward in a random way, but with known probabilities.
In the epidemic context, "forward" corresponds to the crea-
tion of another infective, while "backward" is the identification and isolation of one infective. In this model,
clock time is ignored, and the independent variable is an
integer valued index (counter) which increases by one each
time a forward or backward step occurs. Clearly, if the
starting point is known, as well as the (complementary)
probabilities of forward and backward steps, the probability of a given number of forward steps prior to the first
backward step is easy to determine. Although the random
walk model can be employed in other ways, this one will be
adequate for our purposes.

In Section 7, we first use the birth-death stochastic
process again, and then create and solve an alternative
formulation of the epidemic. This third way to model the
epidemic will be called a branching process. A branching
process is still another standard stochastic model.
Typically it is used to describe the development of successive generation of a family. In the epidemic framework,
the "patriarch" of the family is the initial disease importer, his "sons" are those he infects, and so forth
through successive "generations." In this model clock time
is of no importance, and the disease is seen as spreading
like a chain reaction. Each individual has a probability
density for infecting others and a probability density for
being isolated. These are used to generate an outbreak of
the disease, and the outcome of the model is the ultimate
size of the outbreak. Once again, the branching process
formulation can be used to determine other features of the
epidemic, but these will not be needed in the present
study.

4 The Pre-Epidemic Model

Consider a very large population in which nobody has
smallpox. For the sake of simplicity it is assumed that
the total size of the population is constant. Each day a
number of individuals travel to and from areas of the world
in which smallpox is endemic. Let α be the probability
that on any given day at least one of the arriving individuals is infected with smallpox. (We assume that an individual arriving with the disease manifests no visible symptoms -- if the disease were apparent, the individual would
be isolated immediately, and no outbreak of the disease
could occur.) Note that the probability of disease importation depends on factors which are external to the population under study. Specifically, the probability that an
infected person will arrive depends on the worldwide incidence of smallpox and the level of international travel to
regions where the disease is endemic. These rates (and
hence α) are determined outside the present mathematical
model and are treated here as constants.[3]

Perhaps the clearest way to visualize the situation is
as follows. Each day a binary experiment (Bernoulli trial)
is performed, with the possible outcomes (and corresponding
probabilities):

1. Nobody infected with smallpox enters the population -
   this occurs with probability equal to $(1-\alpha)$.

2. Somebody[4] infected with smallpox enters the population
   - this occurs with probability equal to α.

As the binomial experiments of successive days are
independent random events, it follows immediately that the
probability p_r that smallpox is imported on the rth day is

(1) $$p_r = (1-\alpha)^{r-1}\alpha \quad : \; r = 1, \, 2, \, 3, \, \ldots$$

This expression simply says that for r-1 consecutive days no smallpox is imported (with daily probability 1-α) and then on the rth day smallpox is imported (with probability α). Recognizing that p_r is a geometric density, the expected number of days to the arrival of an infected individual can be easily found to be (See Exercise 3):

(2) $$E\{r\} = \sum_{r=1}^{\infty} r \, p_r = 1/\alpha.$$

This expression allows the quantity α to be estimated from the observed interval between subsequent outbreaks of the disease. Since the expected time between subsequent disease importations is $E\{r\}$, $1/\alpha$ estimates this average time interval.

Assume that during the r days until importation of the disease, individuals are being vaccinated at a rate that leaves a fraction s ($0 \leq s \leq 1$) of the population susceptible to smallpox, and hence a fraction 1-s of the population immune. Since the period of immunity associated with a smallpox vaccination is finite, and since births and immigrants continue to replace deaths and emmigrants in the population, then vaccinations must be done continually in order to maintain the susceptible fraction at the level of s.

Assume that the average number of vaccinations per day in the population is given by V. Associated with each vaccination is a very small risk of death from the vaccination. Let β be the probability of death due to a vaccination, a quantity which will be treated as a constant.[5] During the r days prior to the importation of smallpox, a total of rV vaccinations will be given. Since the outcome of each vaccination is independent of the outcomes of all of the rest, each of the rV vaccinations can be considered as a Bernoulli trial with probability β of death. It then follows that the conditional probability of exactly m deaths, given that the disease is not imported until the rth day, is given by the binomial density which takes the form

(3) $$\text{Prob}\{m|r\} = \binom{rV}{m} \beta^m (1-\beta)^{rV-m}.$$

The quantity sought at this point is the number $E\{m\}$ of deaths caused by the vaccine before the arrival of a single infected individual. This quantity is not immediately available. It is first necessary to calculate the conditional number of deaths prior to the importation of smallpox, given that smallpox is imported on the rth day. This is easily found (See Exercise 4) from (3) to be

$$(4) \qquad E\{m|r\} = \sum_{m=0}^{rV} m \ Prob\{m|r\} = \beta rV.$$

Using (1) to eliminate the conditioning on the number of days r until the importation of smallpox then yields the expected number of vaccine caused deaths as

$$(5) \qquad E\{m\} = \sum_{r=1}^{\infty} E\{m|r\} \ p_r = \sum_{r=1}^{\infty} \beta rV p_r = \beta V \sum_{r=1}^{\infty} r p_r.$$

But this summation was done in equation (2) and yields the result

$$(6) \qquad E\{m\} = \frac{\beta V}{\alpha}.$$

(Readers who are not familiar with the conditional expectation for discrete random variables will find a brief introduction to it in Appendix A.)

Equation (6) relates the expected number of vaccine-caused deaths to the rate constants α and β and to the average daily vaccination rate V. But V is not a simple constant; it is related to the fraction s of the population which is susceptible to smallpox.

We now develop an explicit relationship between V and s, subject to certain simplifying assumptions. Since the total population size, N, has been assumed constant, the total number of individuals who die and emigrate must just exactly be replaced by newborns and immigrants. For simplicity, assume that the fraction dying or emigrating is independent of vaccination status. Thus, among those who die or leave, the fraction susceptible to smallpox is the same as in the general population. Since none of the deaths at this point are due to smallpox, this is a rather reasonable assumption. Assume further that all newborns and immigrants start without smallpox immunity. This is accurate for the newborns but not so good for the immigrants. However, since the total number of immigrants in any year is a small fraction of the total population size, the error introduced by this assumption will be inconsequential.

Let ℓ be the mean survival rate per individual per year for the population, given as a fraction, where "survival" will be understood to mean being alive and still present, and "non-survival" will indicate either death or departure. The fraction of the population which dies or departs each year is therefore given by $1-\ell$. As mentioned earlier, since deaths in the population do not result from smallpox, it is assumed that the proportions of susceptible and immune individuals in the part of the population which dies or departs each year is the same as the proportions in the total population. Recalling that the total population size is N, with a fraction s susceptible and a fraction 1-s immune to smallpox, leads to the partition in Table 2 after one year.

Table 2

	Initially Susceptible	Initially Immune
survive one year	$Ns\ell$	$N(1-s)\ell$
die or depart during year	$Ns(1-\ell)$	$N(1-s)(1-\ell)$

Our present goal is still to derive a relationship that indicates the vaccination rate required to keep the smallpox-susceptible portion of the population fixed at s. There are two naturally occurring effects that tend to increase the susceptible proportion of the population. First, some individuals die or leave the population and are replaced by an equal number of newborns and immigrants, who are assumed to be without any immunity. The size of this group is $N(1-\ell)$. If the proportions of susceptible and immune individuals in the population is to be maintained, a fraction (1 - s) of these new people must be vaccinated. Hence a total of $N(1-\ell)(1-s)$ vaccinations are necessary to offset the effects of death and departure. The second effect that tends naturally to lead to a totally susceptible population is that the immunity resulting from a vaccination lasts only for a finite period of time. For simplicity, assume that a vaccinated individual remains immune for a period of k years.[6] Consequently, of the $N(1-s)\ell$ individuals who are initially immune and who survive for a year, a fraction 1/k would be due for routine revaccination.

Combining the two vaccination quotas above provides the average annual number of vaccinations to maintain the level of susceptibility at s. Division by 365 provides the daily rate as

(7) $$V(s) = [N(1-s)(1-\ell) + N(1-s)\ell/k]/365$$
$$= N(1-s)[1-\ell+\ell/k]/365.$$

By substitution of (7) into (6), we can determine the expected number of deaths that occur prior to the outbreak of a smallpox epidemic and are due to a vaccination program which is designed to maintain the fraction of susceptible individuals at the prescribed level. This completes the model of the first stage of the smallpox outbreak.

5 The Epidemic Initiation Model

The epidemic begins with the arrival in a disease-free area of an individual infected with smallpox, but not yet manifesting any symptoms. The infective arrives unnoticed and unknowingly transmits the disease to others; hence initially the epidemic grows out of control. Before too long, however, one or another of the infected individuals shows symptoms and is diagnosed as a carrier of smallpox. Once the disease is discovered, the initial phase of the epidemic is over.

Since the average time to discovery of the disease is quite short for smallpox, it is reasonable to assume that only a small number of people become infected during the initial phase of the epidemic, even though the number of susceptible individuals in the population may be very large. In addition, it is convenient to assume that the length of the contagious but asymptomatic period (called the incubation period) for each unidentified infective is exponentially distributed. (Readers who are not familiar with Poisson processes and exponentially distributed events should read Appendix B.) Assume also that infectives are identified as having smallpox as soon as symptoms appear.

These assumptions suggest modeling the initial phase of the epidemic as a birth-death stochastic process. To do so, we begin by introducing a random variable, $Y(t)$, whose non-negative integer values represent the number of unidentified cases of smallpox in the population. The disease importer starts the process with $Y(0)=1$.

If it is assumed that at time t there are $Y(t)$ unidentified infectives, then during the next short interval of time, Δt, one of three mutually exclusive things will happen:

1. A susceptible individual can be infected

2. An unidentified infective can be identified

3. Neither a new infection nor an identification occurs.[7]

The probability of one additional undetected case of smallpox (a "birth") depends upon three factors: the number of susceptible individuals in the population, the number of unidentified infectives and a rate constant, λ, which measures the probability of disease transmission per unit time per infective per susceptible. Numerical values of λ are somewhat obscure, but depend upon both natural contagion and social customs. (Do people bow, shake hands or embrace upon meeting one another?) Since it has been assumed that the total population size, N, is very large while the number of infectives, $Y(t)$, is small, the number of susceptible individuals at time t will be approximated by $n=sN$, a constant. An exact specification would subtract $Y(t)$ from n to account for the fact that an individual can not contract the disease more than once during the outbreak of the epidemic. Combining the above quantities leads to an expression for the probability of one additional unidentified case of smallpox during a small time interval Δt if there are $Y(t)$ unidentified cases at time t:

(8a) $\qquad \text{Prob}\{Y \rightarrow Y+1\} = \lambda n Y(t) \Delta t.$

Given our assumption that the length of the incubation period is exponentially distributed, it follows that each of the $Y(t)$ unidentified infectives is as likely as any other to be the first to show external symptoms of small-pox. (Appendix B contains a discussion of equally likely events and exponentially distributed inter-event times). If the expected waiting time for the first appearance of external symptoms is taken to be $1/\omega$, then ω is the probability of symptom manifestation per unit time per unidentified infective (see Exercise 5). Thus the probability that one of the $Y(t)$ infectives will be identified (a "death") during the short interval of time Δt is:

(8b) $\qquad \text{Prob}\{Y \rightarrow Y-1\} = \omega Y(t) \Delta t.$

Note that this quantity does not depend upon the number of susceptible individuals.

It is also possible that during the time interval Δt neither a new unidentified case ("birth") nor an identification ("death") takes place. It therefore follows from (8a) and (8b) that the probability of neither a new unidentified case nor an identification is given by

(8c) $\text{Prob}\{Y \rightarrow Y\} = 1 - \lambda n Y(t) \Delta t - \omega Y(t) \Delta t.$

At this point we could set up a differential-difference equation for the probability that there are Y(t) unidentified infectives at time t (see Exercise 6), but this is not the desired result for the inital phase of the epidemic. What is actually wanted is the expected number, $E\{Y\}$, of unidentified infectives in the population at the instant when the first case manifests external symptoms and thus is identified. This quantity can be easily calculated once it is recognized that the time dependent birth-death process can be reformulated as a simple random walk process which is independent of explicit clock time. All we need do is treat the number of transitions ("births" or "deaths") as the independent variable. Each time a transition occurs, the number of unidentifed infectives either increases or decreases by one. Conveniently, the situation described in (8c) is of no concern for the random walk specification, since it describes a non-transition.

The transition probabilities for the random walk follow directly from a renormalization (scaling so that the probabilities of all available outcomes sum to one) of (8a) and (8b). Since the only types of transition possible are an additional susceptible individual becoming an unidentified infective and an unidentified infective being identified, the probabilities for these events are easily seen to be:

(9a) $\text{Prob}\{\text{additional infective}\} = \dfrac{\lambda n Y(t) \Delta t}{\lambda n Y(t) \Delta t + \omega Y(t) \Delta t}$

$$= \dfrac{\lambda n}{\lambda n + \omega}$$

(9b) $\text{Prob}\{\text{Identification}\} = \dfrac{\omega Y(t) \Delta t}{\lambda n Y(t) \Delta t + \omega Y(t) \Delta t}$

$$= \dfrac{\omega}{\lambda n + \omega}.$$

Since these two events are mutually exclusive and exhaustive, their probabilities sum to unity. Notice also that in renormalization of transition probabilities, explicit dependence on both Y(t) and Δt is eliminated.

It is now a straightforward procedure to find the desired result for the initiation of the epidemic. The probability, P_y, that there are y-1 additional unidentified infectives beyond the initial one (thus that there are Y = y unidentified infectives) followed by the identification of one of these infectives is

(10) $P_y = \left(\dfrac{\lambda n}{\lambda n + \omega}\right)^{y-1} \left(\dfrac{\omega}{\lambda n + \omega}\right).$

Note that (just as in Equation 1) this is a geometric density, hence the expected value of Y is

$$(11) \qquad E\{Y\} = \sum_{y=1}^{\infty} y \, P_y = \frac{\lambda n + \omega}{\omega}.$$

At this point in the epidemic there are $y - 1$ unidentified infectives and one identified case. By actions such as contact tracing and isolation of suspected infectives, the epidemic is brought under control. This final phase of the epidemic is the subject of the next section.

6 The Epidemic Subsidence Model

Once the presence of smallpox in a previously disease-free region is recognized, a concerted effort is made to bring the epidemic to an end. It should however be realized that awareness of the disease and effort at its control, no matter how conscientious, do not reduce the basic contagiousness of the disease. What is changed is the rate at which infectives are identified and isolated from further contact with susceptible individuals. The result is that the total number of individuals infected over time will continue to grow, but the removal rate will increase so as to exceed the infection rate, and consequently the epidemic will eventually die out. The purpose of the epidemic subsidence model is to predict the total number of individuals who contract smallpox before the epidemic runs its course. Two versions of the epidemic subsidence model will be presented. Although these models are formally very different, they lead to identical results. It is instructive to see both as they graphically demonstrate that there is not a single "right way" to formulate the mathematical model.

In developing the first version of the epidemic subsidence model great care must be exercised to avoid confusion. Two intimately related random quantities must be considered. The first, $Y(t)$, which represents the number of unidentified infectives at time t, is the same variable as in the model in the previous section. If the time origin is now set so that $t=0$ is the time when the first infective is identified and isolated (hence the time when the epidemic subsidence model takes over from the epidemic initiation model) it then follows that $Y(0+) = y-1$. (Note

that the quantity found in (11) is the expected value of
$Y(0-)=y$.) As time passes, since the epidemic dies out,
$Y(t)$ shows a generally downward trend. The epidemic is
over when $Y(t)=0$. The second random variable, $Z(t)$, represents the total number of individuals beyond the initial
infective (who imports the disease) who contract smallpox
during the course of the epidemic. It follows that at time
$t=0+$, $Z(0+)=y-1$. Since $Z(t)$ counts cumulative infectives,
it never decreases, and it reaches its maximum value when
the epidemic is over. It is this maximum value which must
be determined.

The first mathematical model for the subsidence of the
epidemic will be based upon the deterministic relationship
between $Y(t)$ and $Z(t)$. Specifically, whenever a new individual contracts smallpox, both $Y(t)$ and $Z(t)$ increase by
one. Whenever a case is identified and isolated, $Y(t)$ decreases by one, but $Z(t)$ is unaffected. Since the probability of an additional infective and also the probability
of identifying an infective will depend upon the number of
unidentified infectives at time t, it is necessary to calculate $Y(t)$, even though the desired result of the model is
to find $Z(t)$ (or more precisely, the expected maximum value
$Z(t)$ achieves).

As was true with the epidemic initiation models, the
subsidence model must recognize three distinct situations.
The first of these corresponds to development of a new case
of smallpox in a susceptible individual. By (8a) in the
previous section, and by the definition of $Y(t)$ and $Z(t)$,
we have

(12a) $\text{Prob}\{Y \rightarrow Y+1 \ \& \ Z \rightarrow Z+1\} = \lambda n Y(t) \Delta t.$

The second situation corresponds to removal of an infective
from contact with susceptible individuals. Since this may
well occur prior to the development of any externally observable symptoms (purely as a result of conscientious public health measures) the removal rate will be faster than
during the initiation phase of the epidemic. Formally,
this amounts to nothing more than replacing ω by μ (where
$\mu \gg \omega$) in (8b) and including both $Y(t)$ and $Z(t)$ in the
definition:

(12b) $\text{Prob}\{Y \rightarrow Y-1 \ \& \ Z \rightarrow Z\} = \mu Y(t) \Delta t.$

Note that as mentioned earlier, although $Y(t)$ decreases
when a case is isolated, $Z(t)$ does not change. In the
third and only other situation, neither a new case nor a
removal occurs in the short time interval Δt. Following
(8c), we have

(12c) $\text{Prob}\{Y \rightarrow Y \ \& \ Z \rightarrow Z\} = 1 - \lambda n Y(t) \Delta t - \mu Y(t) \Delta t.$

Developing an equation for the behavior of the quantity

(13) $p_{y,z}(t) = \text{Prob}\{Y(t)=y, Z(t)=z\}$

is now a straightforward procedure. To do it, consider the
quantity $p_{y,z}(t+\Delta t)$, and recognize that it can arise only
in three mutually exclusive ways:

1.   at time t there are y-1 unidentified and z-1 cumulative
     infectives with probability $p_{y-1,z-1}(t)$, and during the
     next Δt of time another case develops with probability
     from (12a) of $\lambda n(y-1)\Delta t$

2.   at time t there are y+1 unidentified and z cumulative
     infectives with probability $p_{y+1,z}(t)$, and during the
     next Δt of time another case is isolated with probabil-
     ity from (12b) of $\mu(y+1)\Delta t$

3.   at time t there are y unidentified and z cumulative in-
     fectives with probability $p_{y,z}(t)$, and during the next
     Δt of time there is neither another case developed nor
     one isolated. By (12c), this occurs with probability
     $1 - \lambda n y \Delta t - \mu y \Delta t$.

Combining these three situations leads to the relation

(14)

$$p_{y,z}(t+\Delta t) = [\lambda n(y-1)\Delta t]p_{y-1,z-1}(t)$$
$$+ [\mu(y+1)\Delta t]p_{y+1,z}(t)$$
$$+ [1 - \lambda n y \Delta t - \mu y \Delta t]p_{y,z}(t).$$

Upon rearranging, dividing through by Δt and letting $\Delta t \to 0$,
we obtain the governing equation for the subsidence of the
epidemic:

(15)

$$\frac{d}{dt} p_{y,z}(t) = \lambda n(y-1)p_{y-1,z-1}(t) - (\lambda n+\mu)y p_{y,z}(t)$$
$$+ \mu(y+1)p_{y+1,z}(t)$$

Equation (15) is a differential-difference equation for the
joint probability density $p_{y,z}(t)$. From the facts that
$Y(0+)=y-1$ and $Z(0+)=y-1$, it follows that $p_{y-1,y-1}(0+)=1$.
     This differential-difference equation will now be used
to determine how the epidemic proceeds. While it would be
possible (at least in theory) to find $p_{y,z}(t)$, what is
really wanted is the expected value of $Z(t)$ at the end of
the epidemic; hence we consider

(16a) $E\{Y(t)\} = \sum_{y=0}^{\infty} \sum_{z=0}^{\infty} y\, p_{y,z}(t)$

(16b) $E\{Z(t)\} = \sum_{y=0}^{\infty} \sum_{z=0}^{\infty} z\, p_{y,z}(t).$

In order to continue, differentiate these expressions with respect to time to get

$$(17) \qquad \frac{d}{dt} E\{Y(t)\} = \sum_{y=0}^{\infty} \sum_{z=0}^{\infty} y \frac{d}{dt} P_{y,z}(t)$$

from (16a) and an analogous expression from (16b), and substitute the expression for the derivative on the right-hand side from (15). After a straightforward but lengthy bit of algebra which involves using the definitions (16a) and (16b) to carry out the summations (see Exercise 7), the following pair of coupled differential equations results

$$(18a) \qquad \frac{d}{dt} E\{Y(t)\} = (\lambda n - \omega) E\{Y(t)\}$$

$$(18b) \qquad \frac{d}{dt} E\{Z(t)\} = \lambda n E\{Y(t)\}.$$

Fortunately, these equations are very easy to solve. Notice that the first equation does not involve $E\{Z(t)\}$ and hence can be solved by itself. Equation (18a) is a first order differential equation that can be solved either by separation of variables or by treating it as a linear differential equation; in any case the solution is:

$$(19) \qquad E\{Y(t)\} = E\{Y(0+)\} e^{(\lambda n - \mu) t}$$

where $E\{Y(0+)\}$ is the number of unidentified infectives just after the first case of smallpox is identified. This quantity was found earlier in the epidemic initiation model (see Equation 11). Note that since it has been assumed that the epidemic will die out, it follows that $E\{Y(t)\} \to 0$ as $t \to \infty$, thus we must have $\lambda n < \mu$.

The next step is to solve (18b) for $E\{Z(t)\}$. This is easy to do since the right-hand side is now a known function of time from (19). Substitution from (19), multiplying through by dt and integrating formally leads to

$$(20) \qquad E\{Z(t)\} = E\{Y(0+)\} \frac{\lambda n}{\lambda n - \mu} e^{(\lambda n - \mu) t} + K$$

where K is a constant of integration. This constant is evaluated by setting t=0+ in (20) and using the relation $E\{Z(0+)\} = E\{Y(0+)\}$, so that

$$(21) \qquad K = \frac{\mu}{\mu - \lambda n} E\{Y(0+)\}.$$

The result that is sought is the maximum value for $E\{Z(t)\}$, which represents the expected number of cases of smallpox (beyond the initial, imported case) that occur during the epidemic. Since the epidemic is certain to die out, the maximum value of $E\{Z(t)\}$ may be found by letting $t \to \infty$ in

(20). But since $\lambda n < \mu$, the exponential in (20) goes to zero; thus

(22) $$\lim_{t \to \infty} E\{Z(t)\} = K = \frac{\mu}{\mu - \lambda n} E\{Y(0+)\}$$

where K is known from (21).

This completes the formulation and solution of the first version of the epidemic subsidence model. Notice that the model describes the development of the epidemic as a function of time, but without any regard for the pattern of contagion. The second version of the model results from the observation that all infectives except the disease importer contract the disease from someone who already has it. At the time when the epidemic subsidence model takes effect, the expected number of unidentified infectives is known. Each of these may infect susceptibles before being identified and isolated, and the newly infected individuals repeat the process. The consequence is that the epidemic

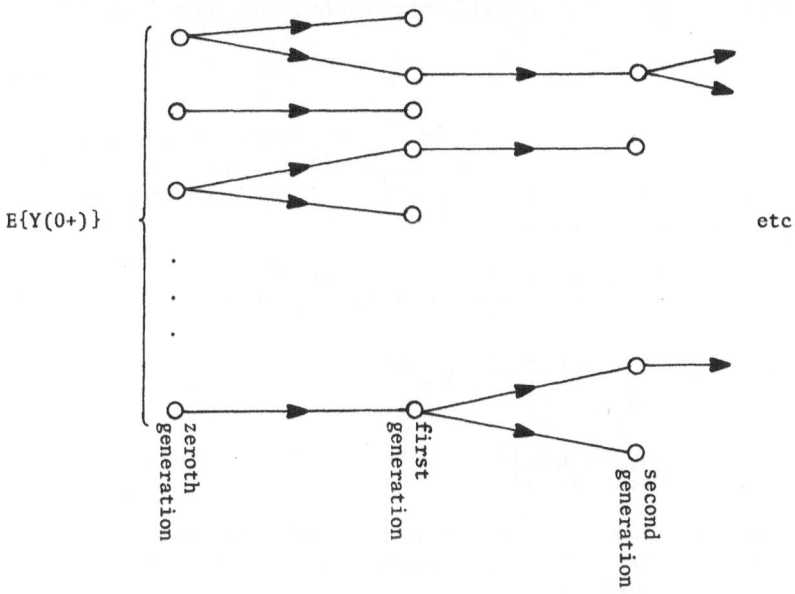

Figure 1. The subsidence phase of a typical epidemic viewed as a branching process.

subsidence phase can be described by a directed graph whose vertices represent infectives and whose edges are directed from disease source to disease recipient as illustrated in Figure 1. It is convenient to think of the $E\{Y(0+)\}$ individuals present when the model begins as the zeroth generation, the people they infect as the first generation, and so forth until the epidemic ends. The stochastic model which describes this way of visualizing the epidemic is called a branching process. We proceed next to develop this model.

Consider one of the unidentified infectives present when the first case of smallpox is recognized and isolated. It has been assumed that the probability of discovery and removal from circulation at time t is exponentially distributed with parameter μ, thus

(23) $\text{Prob}\{\text{removal at time t}\} = \mu e^{-\mu t}$.

Until the disease is discovered, the unidentified infective in question is potentially spreading smallpox to susceptibles. The disease is spread at random; as noted before, the number of cases transmitted per individual infective per unit time is λn. Thus, if the infective circulates spreading smallpox for time t, it follows (see Appendix B) that

$$\text{Prob}\left\{\begin{array}{l}\text{one infective transmits}\\\text{disease to j susceptibles}\end{array}\middle|\begin{array}{l}\text{that infective remains}\\\text{unidentified for time t}\end{array}\right\}$$

(24) $= \dfrac{(\lambda nt)^j\, e^{-\lambda nt}}{j!}$

which is a Poisson distribution. To eliminate the time conditioning, multiply by the probability that the infective remains unidentified for time t from (23) and integrate with respect to time; thus

$$P_j = \text{Prob}\left\{\begin{array}{l}\text{one infective transmits}\\\text{disease to j susceptibles}\end{array}\right\}$$

$$= \int_0^\infty \dfrac{(\mu nt)\, e^{-\lambda nt}}{j!}\, \mu e^{-\mu t}\, dt$$

(25) $= \dfrac{\mu}{n\lambda + \mu}\left(\dfrac{n\lambda}{n\lambda + \mu}\right)^j$

a result which follows from repeated integration by parts (see Exercise 8). The expected number of new cases, θ, caused by one infective is

(26) $\theta = \displaystyle\sum_{j=0}^{\infty} j\, P_j = \dfrac{n\lambda}{\mu}$.

As noted earlier, $\mu > \lambda n$, hence $\theta < 1$.

We must next design the model for the branching process. This model will extend the results just determined for one infective to the whole epidemic. Assume that the number of cases of the disease transmitted by each infective is independent of the number transmitted by any other infective, and that the probability, P_j, from (25) of transmitting j cases is the same for each infective. Let U_i be the integer valued random variable that counts the number of new infectives created by the ith individual infective; it follows from (26) that

(27) $E\{U_i\} = \theta$.

Also, let W_m be an integer valued random variable that counts the total number of infectives in the mth disease generation that follow from one particular infective in the zeroth generation. Since by this definition there are W_{m-1} infectives in the $m-1^{st}$ disease generation, we have

(28) $W_m = \sum_{i=1}^{W_{m-1}} U_i$.

The expected value of W_m follows easily from the conditional expectation given W_{m-1}; thus

$$E\{W_m\} = E\{E[W_m|W_{m-1}]\}$$

(29a) $= E\{E[\sum_{i=1}^{W_{m-1}} U_i|W_{m-1}]\}$.

By equation (28) for W_m, and since the expectation of the sum equals the sum of the expectations, we have

(29b) $E\{W_m\} = E\{\sum_{i=1}^{W_{m-1}} E(U_i)|W_{m-1}\}$.

Substituting θ for $E(U_i)$ by (27) and carrying out the summation yields

(29c) $E\{W_m\} = E\{\theta W_{m-1}\}$.

This is a simple difference equation which can be solved (see Exercise 9) by using induction and the fact that $E\{W_0\}$ =1 (since the model counts the infectives that develop from a single infective in the zeroth generation); we find

(30) $E\{W_m\} = \theta^m$.

The total number, Z, of cases involved in the epidemic is then just the product of the number in the zeroth generation times the sum of the number in each generation resulting from each infective in the zeroth generation

(31) $Z = Y(0+) \sum_{m=0}^{\infty} \theta^m = \dfrac{Y(0+)}{1-\theta}$.

-25-

The expected number of cases of smallpox in the entire epidemic is then

$$(32) \qquad E\{Z\} = \frac{E\{Y(0+)\}}{1-\theta} = \frac{\mu}{\mu-\lambda n} E\{Y(0+)\}.$$

which agrees with the result found earlier using the multi-process model.

All that remains is to put the models for the three phases of the epidemic together in order to answer the question of the optimum level of vaccination to minimize total deaths.

7 The Optimal Vaccination Policy

Since for the past 30 years outbreaks of smallpox have occurred infrequently in most parts of the developed world, it seems reasonable to seek that level of vaccine-induced immunity which minimizes the average number of deaths that would occur between the ends of two successive epidemics. This amounts to choosing the level of susceptibility s in a population so that the average number of deaths which occur during one (long) period when there is no disease present and the subsequent (short) period of epidemic is a minimum.

Note that the process of optimization consists of trading one cause of death for another. If the fraction, s, of the population which is susceptible to smallpox is made small by extensive vaccination, then epidemic-caused deaths are traded for vaccine-caused deaths. If instead s is allowed to become large by reducing the vaccination rate, vaccine-caused deaths are traded for epidemic-caused deaths. It should be realized that the optimal value of s might turn out to be s=0 (vaccinate everybody) or s=1 (vaccinate nobody) or some intermediate value, 0<s<1.

In order to proceed, it is necessary to establish the expected number of vaccine- and epidemic-caused deaths as a function of the susceptibility, s. These quantities are easily found from the three stage mathematical model. The expected number of vaccine caused deaths, $D_v(s)$, is given in (6), with V=V(s) found from (7); hence

$$(33) \qquad D_v(s) = \frac{\beta N}{\alpha} \; \frac{1 - \ell + \ell/k}{365} \; (1-s).$$

Note that $D_v(s)$ is simply a linearly decreasing function of s which goes to zero when s=1 (no vaccination). The ex-

-27-

pected number of epidemic-caused deaths, $D_e(s)$, can be found by combining the results of the epidemic initiation and subsidence models. The expected number of smallpox cases (beyond the initial importer) is given by Equation (22) or (32). The expected total number of cases (including the initial importer) is therefore

$$(34) \quad E\{\text{total cases}\} = 1 + \frac{\mu}{\mu - \lambda n} E\{Y(0+)\}.$$

The fact that $E\{Y(0+)\}$ is the expected number of unidentified infectives in the population after the first case is discovered provides the connection with the epidemic initiation model. It is apparent immediately that

$$(35) \quad E\{Y(0+)\} = E\{Y\} - 1 = \frac{\lambda n}{\omega}$$

where $E\{Y\}$ is the expected number of unidentified cases of smallpox just prior to the first discovery of the disease, which was found in (11). Substituting (35) into (34) and using $n=sN$ yields the expected number of total cases of smallpox in the epidemic as a function of the susceptibility level. If a fraction ν of all cases are fatal, the expected number of epidemic deaths is

$$(36) \qquad D_e(s) = \nu \left[1 + \frac{\mu \lambda Ns}{\omega(\mu - \lambda Ns)} \right].$$

Notice that $D_e(s)$ increases as s increases. If $s=0$, the entire population is immune, and the disease importer (who is the only one to contract smallpox) dies with probability equal to ν. As the susceptible fraction of the population increases, the number of epidemic deaths rises at a faster than linear rate. (To understand this, observe that the increase would be linear if s did not appear in the denominator of the second term in the square brackets. Since s does in fact appear in the denominator in such a way that the denominator decreases with increasing s, the rise in mortality is faster than linear.) Note further that since $\mu > \lambda Ns = \lambda n$ (the condition which guarantees that the epidemic dies out), the denominator is always positive (as it must be for (36) to make physical sense).

During one complete epidemic cycle, which includes the pre-epidemic period, the initial outbreak and the subsequent remission of the disease, the expected total number of deaths, $D(s)$, is simply the sum of the vaccination and epidemic-caused deaths; hence

$$(37) \qquad D(s) = D_v(s) + D_e(s)$$

where $D_v(s)$ is given in (33) and $D_e(s)$ in (36). The next problem is to find an expression for the value of s that minimizes D(s) for $0 \leq s \leq 1$. This is a simple exercise in calculus (see Exercise 10). The value of s=s* that minimizes D(s) can be found by differentiating D(s) with respect to s and setting the result equal to zero. (Note that this procedure could equally well yield a maximum, but on physical grounds no such maximum makes sense. This assertion can be confirmed by determining the sign of the second derivative of D(s) with respect to s at s=s*.)

The minimization procedure described above leads easily to the following result:

$$(38) \qquad s^* = \frac{\mu}{\lambda N} \left[1 - \frac{365\alpha\lambda\nu}{\omega\beta[1-\ell+\ell/k]} \right]^{1/2}$$

And from (38) it follows that

$$(39a) \qquad s^* = 0; \text{ if } 365\alpha\lambda\nu \geq \omega\beta[1-\ell+\ell/k]$$

$$(39b) \quad s^* = \min\left\{ \frac{\mu}{\lambda N} \left[1 - \frac{365\alpha\lambda\nu}{\omega\beta[1-\ell+\ell/k]} \right]^{1/2} , 1 \right\}; \text{other-wise}$$

This completes the general solution to the problem. To apply this solution in practice, we must estimate the values of the various parameters in Equations (39), and then determine the appropriate choice of s=s*. Once this choice is made, the appropriate vaccination rate V=V(s*) can be found from (7).

8 Calibrating the Model

Estimating the values of the parameters in (39) is a non-trivial task. One might argue that extensive amounts of data and sophisticated statistical procedures should be employed. However, since the mathematical model is at best approximate, rough estimates are apt to be adequate. The results should permit authorities to decide whether the model implies that vaccination should unequivocally be discontinued (s=1), or enthusiastically pursued (s=0), or that some intermediate course of action should be followed. With all the detail that has been omitted from the model, it is inappropriate to quote a value of s* to three decimal places.

Rough estimates for the parameters relevant to the United States in the 1950's are listed below, along with brief explanations (see Bailey, 1975).

$\alpha = 10^{-3}$: Since $1/\alpha$ is the expected waiting time for disease importation, this estimate implies a mean inter-epidemic period of 1000 days, or just under three years. If the waiting time were longer, this estimate would tend to bias results so as to favor higher vaccination rates.

$\beta = 10^{-6}$: In the data cited in Section 1 for the United States in 1968, 9 individuals died when 14 million were vaccinated. Hence we assume that about one vaccination in a million leads to complications that result in death.

$\ell = 0.99$: In the United States each year about one person in a hundred dies, hence 99 out of one hundred survive for a year.

k = 4: Ordinarily, revaccination is required every 3 - 5
years to maintain immunity. Choosing k=4 represents a
compromise.

$N = 2 \times 10^8$: The total population of the United States for
the past 30 years has been roughly 200 million people.

$\omega = 0.2$: Since $1/\omega$ is the expected waiting time to discovery of the first case of smallpox, this choice implies
that it will take 5 days for the epidemic to be de-
tected.

$\mu = 2.0$: With conscientious contact tracing, the removal
rate for infectives can be made an order of magnitude
larger than ω, the removal rate prior to the detection
of the disease. With $\mu=2$, infectives would spend only
one half day (average time) before being isolated from
further contact with susceptibles.

$\nu = 10^{-1}$: About one person in ten who contracts smallpox
subsequently dies of the disease.

λ The disease transmission rate will not be assigned a
particular value but will instead be retained as a
parameter. For some intuitive meaning, recall that if
the entire population were susceptible, then on average
each infective would cause λN new cases of smallpox
each day. Consequently, λN is probably somewhere between one and two for the United States. As further
justification, recall that for the epidemic to subside,
$\lambda n < \mu$. If the model suggests that s=1 (no vaccination),
then $\lambda N < \mu$ implies $\lambda N < 2$. (It should be realized that
this last argument is included as a consistency check
only.)

The estimates of s* which result from substituting
these values for the parameters into (39) are shown in
Figure 2 as a function of λN. Notice that the model suggests that vaccination should be entirely discontinued if
$\lambda N < 1.84$, while if $\lambda N > 282$, the entire population should be
vaccinated. Since the most realistic range of values for
the disease transmission rate is roughly $1 \leq \lambda N \leq 2$, the impli-
cation is that vaccination can be prudently reduced to a
very low level without serious risk. In fact, since by
about 1955 the choice of α could already have been seen as
tending to overestimate the desirability of vaccination in
the United States, it seems reasonable to say that the
model would have supported a change in policy at that time,
to require only that persons entering from abroad (and pos-
sibly hospital workers) be vaccinated.

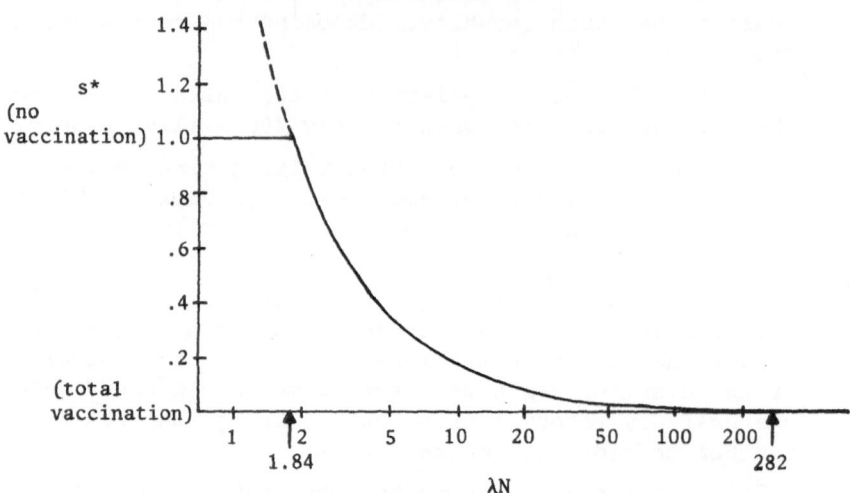

Figure 2. Optimal level of Susceptibility s* so as to minimize
expected total deaths due to the combined effects of
vaccination and epidemic as a function of the disease
transmission parameter, λN.

9 Concluding Remarks

In light of the apparent worldwide eradication of smallpox, one might reasonably ask whether the models just discussed have any real significance. The answer is emphatically yes. For further application, we note that there are other diseases for which there is a prevention but no cure. The basic ideas if not the precise details of the models might apply, for example, to poliomyelitis, influenza, or measles. History has shown that if the quantitative approach had been applied to smallpox vaccination policy in the United States or Western Europe twenty years ago, it might have led to a substantial decrease in the waste of human and monetary resources on unnecessary vaccinations. Obviously no one would seriously consider making a $150 million a year decision based on the results of models at the simplified level of our prototypes, even if there were no fatalities involved. Features that should be added to make the models viable as bases for changing public policy include the age structure of the population, the difference in mortality rates between the first and subsequent vaccinations, and the different exposure risks to various population subgroups.

One final irony deserves mention. Although smallpox has been declared dead, there are presently samples of the virus in at least six laboratories throughout the world, saved for experimental purposes. Our models provide a reasonable recommendation to reasonable people; we must now hope that there will be no serious failures of laboratory precautions and no use of viral warfare to bring back this hideous disease.

Bibliography

Bailey, N.T.J., 1975, <u>The Mathematical Theory of Infectious Diseases</u>, Chapter 20, Hafner Press, New York.

Becker, N., 1972, "Vaccination Programmes for Rare Infectious Diseases," <u>Biometrika</u>, Vol. 59, No. 2, pp.443-453.

Bernoulli, D., 1760, "Essai d'une nouvelle analyse de la mortalité causée par la petite vérole et des avantages de l'inoculation pour la prévenir," <u>Mem. Math. Phys. Acad. Roy. Sci.</u>, Paris, pp.1-45.

Bradley, L., 1971, <u>Smallpox Inoculation: An Eighteenth Century Mathematical Controversy</u>, Adult Education Department, University of Nottingham.

Breman, J.G., and Arita, I., 1980, "The Confirmation and Maintenance of Smallpox Eradication," <u>New England Journal of Medicine</u>, Vol. 303, No. 22, pp. 1263-1272.

Brown, G.C. (ed.), 1971, "Is Routine Smallpox Vaccination Necessary in the United States?" A Symposium, <u>American Journal of Epidemiology</u>, Vol. 93, No. 4, pp. 222-252. (The symposium consists of the following papers:)

   Brown, G.C., "Introduction"

   Foege, W.H., Foster, S.O. and Goldstein, J.A., "Current Status of Global Smallpox Eradication."

   Gelfand, H.M. and Posch, J., "The Recent Outbreak of Smallpox in Meschede, West Germany."

Lane, J.M. and Miller, J.D., "Risk of Smallpox Vaccination Complications in the United States."

Katz, S.L., "The Case for Continuing Routine Childhood Smallpox Vaccination in the United States."

Neff, J.M., "The Case for Abolishing Routine Childhood Smallpox Vaccination in the United States."

Benenson, A.S., "Possible Alternatives to Routine Smallpox Vaccination in the United States."

d'Alembert, J.l'R., 1761, Opuscules Mathématiques, Vol. 2.

Geison, G.L., 1978, "The Eradication of Smallpox: a Revisionist View," Science, Vol. 201, pp. 519-520.

Henderson, D.A., 1976, "The Eradication of Smallpox," Scientific American, Vol. 235, No. 4, pp. 25-33.

Lane, J.M., Ruben, F.L., Neff, J.M. and Miller, J.D., 1969, "Complications of Smallpox Vaccination, 1968: National Surveillance in the United States," New England Journal of Medicine, Vol. 281, No. 22, pp. 1201-1208.

Langer, W.L., 1976, "Immunization against Smallpox before Jenner," Scientific American, Vol. 234, No. 1, pp. 112-117.

Razzell, P., 1977, Edward Jenner's Cowpox Vaccine. The History of a Medical Myth. Calaban Books, Firle, Lewes, Sussex, England.

Stockton, William, 1979, "Smallpox is not dead." New York Times, 4 February 1979.

Footnotes

1. A somewhat controversial book has recently been pub-
   lished (Razzell, 1977) in which it is suggested that
   Jenner's famous vaccine against smallpox was not really
   cowpox virus as Jenner thought, but rather an attenu-
   ated strain of smallpox virus. This book is unfortunately rather hard to obtain due to its limited circulation; a fairly detailed description of the content
   can be found in a book review by Geison (1978).

2. Although there is no known reservoir for smallpox, this
   does not prove that none exists. A really basic question is whether smallpox will ever spontaneously recur
   from some unknown reservoir. Epidemiologists are concerned by the fact that certain pox virus species such
   as monkeypox can affect humans and are very similar to
   smallpox, while others (such as whitepox) do not appear
   to affect humans but are otherwise indistinguishable
   from smallpox. For more details about this, see Breman
   and Arita, 1980.

3. In a refined version of the model these rates could
   exhibit both secular trends (the worldwide incidence of
   smallpox was declining while the number of international travellers was increasing) and annual periodicity
   (the incidence of smallpox tended to rise during the
   cold months of the year, while international travel to
   and from the United States is highest in the summer).

4. Strictly speaking, this should not say "somebody" but
   rather "one or more individuals." However, since the
   arrival probability α will turn out to be very small,

the probability that more than one person arrives with smallpox on a given day is so small that it can be ignored (see Exercise 2).

5. It would be preferable to recognize in the model that β depends upon factors such as age, physical condition, whether it is a first vaccination or a revaccination, ... but to include this degree of detail would substantially complicate the model. Ultimately, the greatest risk by far occurs with primary vaccination of very small children. Since this group represents a fairly constant fraction of the total population, treating β as a constant may not be too unreasonable.

6. In reality, the immunity due to a vaccination would die away slowly instead of being totally present or absent. A prudent public health policy would account for this by re-vaccinating at regular intervals (once every k years).

7. By assuming that Δt is small, the possibility of more than one event (new infective or identification) during an interval of length Δt can be made negligibly small. In deriving the birth-death process, Δt will be allowed to approach zero in the limit. The assumption of no more than one event during an interval of length Δt then amounts to saying that no two events occur exactly simultaneously.

APPENDIX A
Conditional Expectations

Consider that two discrete random variables, U and W, assume values u_1, u_2, u_3, ... and w_1, w_2, w_3, ... respectively. The joint density for U and W is defined by:

(A1) $\text{Prob}\{U=u_i, W=w_j\} = P_{UW}(u_i,w_j)$: $i,j = 0, 1, 2, ...$

The marginal densities for U and W are obtained by summation over one or the other of the two indices:

(A2a) $\text{Prob}\{U=u_i\} = \sum_{j=0}^{\infty} P_{UW}(u_i,w_j) = P_U(u_i)$: $i = 0, 1, 2, ...$

(A2b) $\text{Prob}\{W=w_j\} = \sum_{i=0}^{\infty} P_{UW}(u_i,w_j) = P_W(w_j)$: $j = 0, 1, 2, ...$

The conditional density for $W=w_j$ given that $U=u_i$ is then defined by the ratio

(A3) $\text{Prob}\{W=w_j|U=u_i\} = \dfrac{P_{UW}(u_i,w_j)}{P_U(u_i)}$: $i,j = 0, 1, 2, ...$

Note that a similar expression could be defined for the conditional density for $U=u_i$ given that $W=w_j$, but this will not be needed.

The expected value for W is defined by the expression

(A4) $E\{W\} = \sum_{j=0}^{\infty} w_j \, P_W(w_j)$

which by using (A2b) can be rewritten in the form

(A5) $E\{W\} = \sum_{i=0}^{\infty} \sum_{j=0}^{\infty} w_j \, P_{UW}(u_i,w_j)$

and then by (A3) in the form

$$(A6) \quad E\{W\} = \sum_{i=0}^{\infty} \sum_{j=0}^{\infty} w_j \, P_{W|U} \, (w_j|u_i) \, P_U(u_i).$$

The conditional expectation of W given that $U=u_i$ is defined by the expression

$$(A7) \quad E\{W|U=u_i\} = \sum_{j=0}^{\infty} w_j \, P_{W|U} \, (w_j|u_i) : i = 0, 1, 2, \ldots$$

it then follows immediately from (A6) that

$$(A8) \quad E\{W\} = \sum_{i=0}^{\infty} E\{W|U = u_i\} \, P_U \, \{u_i\}.$$

In evaluating $E\{W\}$ it is frequently convenient first to find $E\{W|U=u_i\}$ from (A7) and then to use (A8) to eliminate the conditioning (see Exercise 11).

APPENDIX B
Poisson Processes
and Exponentially Distributed
Events

Let $X(t)$ be an integer valued random variable such that

(B1) $\text{Prob}\{X(t)=n\} = p_n(t); \; n = 0, 1, 2, \ldots$

It is convenient to think of $X(t)$ as a cumulative counter that, starting from some selected time t=0, registers the number of occurrences of some event up to time t. For example, $X(t)$ might be the number of particles emitted by a radioactive source during some interval of observation time.

Assume that the events occur at random; that is, that the occurrence of an event at any particular instant of time does not influence the chance that an event will occur at any other time. Let γ be the rate constant for the random events, which means that the probability that an event occurs in a very short time interval Δt is $\gamma \Delta t$. Consequently, the probability that no event occurs is $(1-\gamma \Delta t)$, and the probability that two or more events occur in the very short interval Δt is negligible.

Suppose we wish to determine $p_n(t+\Delta t)$ for n>0. There are two situations which permit this: either that at time t, $X(t)=n-1$ with probability $p_{n-1}(t)$ and an event occurs during the next interval of length Δt with probability $\gamma \Delta t$, or else that at time t, $X(t)=n$ with probability $p_n(t)$ and no event occurs during the next interval of length Δt with probability $(1-\gamma \Delta t)$. In the form of an equation, this becomes

(B2) $p_n(t+\Delta t) = p_{n-1}(t) \; \gamma \Delta t + p_n(t) \; (1 - \gamma \Delta t).$

Rearranging, and taking the limit as $\Delta t \rightarrow 0$ leads to

(B3a) $\dfrac{dp_n(t)}{dt} = \gamma[p_{n-1}(t) - p_n(t)]: n = 1, 2, \ldots$

If n=0, an arguement like the one above leads to the equation

(B3b) $\dfrac{dp_0(t)}{dt} = -\gamma p_0(t).$

Imagine that we start the random process with $X(0)=0$, so

(B4a) $p_n(0) = 0 \; ; \; n = 1, 2, 3 \ldots$

(B4b) $p_0(0) = 1.$

Equation (B3b) can be solved using separation and integration. The initial condition given in (B4b) then yields

(B5) $p_0(t) = e^{-\gamma t}.$

Next, set n=1 in (B3a) and substitute $p_0(t)$ from (B5) to get

(B6) $\dfrac{dp_1(t)}{dt} + \gamma p_1(t) = \gamma e^{-\gamma t}.$

But if we multiply both sides of (B6) by $e^{\gamma t}$, we obtain

(B7) $d[e^{\gamma t} p_1(t)] = \gamma dt$

which we can integrate directly; with the initial condition (B4a) this yields

(B8) $p_1(t) = \gamma t e^{-\gamma t}.$

Repeating the same procedure which worked for n=1 inductively leads to the general result

(B9) $p_n(t) = \dfrac{(\gamma t)^n \, e^{-\gamma t}}{n!} \; ; \; n = 0, 1, 2, \ldots$

This is the well known time dependent Poisson density function which describes the probability that by time t, exactly n random events have occurred.

Notice next that $p_0(\tau) = e^{-\gamma\tau}$ is the probability that no event has occurred by time $t=\tau$; or in other words, that the first event takes place after time τ. Thus,

(B10) $\qquad F(\tau) = 1 - e^{-\gamma\tau}$

is the distribution function for the occurrence of the first event before time τ, and the derivative

(B11) $\qquad f(\tau) = \dfrac{dF(\tau)}{d\tau} = \gamma e^{-\gamma\tau}$

is the corresponding density function (i.e., the probability that the first event occurs at time τ).

Perhaps the most interesting aspect of this result is that it is independent of where the zero point of time is located. Thus, if $\tau=0$ is chosen to correspond to any particular event, (B11) describes the probability density for the time of occurrence of the next event.

Exercises

1. In 1760 Daniel Bernoulli set up a model allowing him to analyze the effects of inoculation of the number of deaths caused by smallpox. He considered the effects of the disease on one cohort group; that is, of all the individuals born in one specific year.

   Define $N(t)$ to be the number in a cohort group who survived until age t, and $S(t)$ to be the number who have not had the disease by age t and are still susceptible to it. Let p, $0 \leq p \leq 1$ be the probability of a susceptible acquiring the disease and $1/m$, $m \geq 1$ the probability of dying from smallpox once it is acquired. Taking $S(t)$ as a differentiable function, then compute the rate $dS(t)/dt$ at which the number of susceptibles is changing (decreasing) by adding an expression for the rate at which susceptibles at age t are infected to one for the rate of removal of susceptibles due to death from all causes besides smallpox. The resulting equation of Bernoulli is

   $$\frac{dS(t)}{dt} = -pS(t) + \frac{S(t)}{N(t)} \frac{dN(t)}{dt} + pS^2(t)/mN(t).$$

   a. Use the substitution $y=N/S$ to transform this into a solvable differential equation for y: $dy/dt = py - p/m$.

   b. Bernoulli argued on the basis of mortality tables that both p and m were independent of age, hence constant. Assuming this, obtain the following solution

   $$S(t) = mN(t)/[1+(m-1)e^{tp}].$$

c. Bernoulli estimated $p = 1/8$ and $m = 8$ for Paris of the 1760's. Use these estimates to find the proportion of twenty five year olds in one cohort group who would already have had smallpox.

d. Use the same values of p and m as in part c, but assume that one half of the cohort group was innoculated and kept immune essentially since age zero. If the immunized individuals are regarded as survivors of the disease, compute the same proportion as in part c.

e. There are two limiting cases that are of interest: $m \to 1$, that is, the mortality rate is very high, and $m \to \infty$, the mortality rate is very low. Determine what happens to $S(t)/N(t)$ in these cases, and convince yourself that the results are what you should have expected.

2. In the text describing the Pre-Epidemic Model, it is assumed that the daily probability that no disease carrier will arrive is $(1-\alpha)$. Consider one particular day on which M foreign travelers arrive. Assume that each of these travelers has probability ε of being infected with smallpox, and that the likelihood for each is independent of all of the others (probably not a very good assumption since people often travel with family or friends). Assume that M and ε are consistent with an overall daily probability of no disease importer of $(1-\alpha)$. Compare the probability of just one imported case with the probability of exactly two cases on a particular day, assuming for example that $\alpha = .001$ and $M = 1000$.

3. Assuming that the probability, p_r, that the disease is first imported on the rth day is given by $p_r = (1-\alpha)^{r-1}\alpha$, show that the expected waiting time to the first importation is given by $E\{r\}) = 1/\alpha$.

4. If the probability of m vaccine caused deaths given that vaccination is continued for r days is

$$\text{Prob}\{m|r\} = \binom{rV}{m}\beta^m(1-\beta)^{rV-m}$$

show that the conditional expected number of deaths is $E\{m|r\} = \beta rV$.

5. It is claimed in the Epidemic Initiation Model that the length of the incubation period for each infected individual is exponentially distributed with parameter ω. Show that this implies that the expected duration of the incubation period is then $1/\omega$.

6. Starting from the transition probabilities given in Equation (8) and the definition $p_y = \text{Prob}\{Y(t)=y\}$, derive a differential-difference equation for the birth-death process.

-43-

(Hint: study the derivation of the multi-process derived in
the section of the Epidemic Subsidence Model and use an analogous procedure.)

7. Given the definitions in (15) and (16), derive the coupled
    differential equations given in (18).

8. Use repeated integration by parts to show that

$$\int_0^\infty \frac{(\lambda nt)^j\, e^{-\lambda nt}}{j!}\, \mu e^{-\mu t}\, dt = \left(\frac{\mu}{n\lambda+\mu}\right)\left(\frac{n\lambda}{n\lambda+\mu}\right)^j$$

9. Use successive substitution on the difference equation

$$E\{W_m\} = \theta\, E\{W_{m-1}\}$$

with the initial condition $E\{W_0\}=1$, to show that $E\{W_m\}=\theta^m$.

10. Given that

$$D(s) = \frac{\beta N}{\alpha}\ \frac{1-\ell+\ell/k}{365}\ (1-s) + \nu\ \left[1 + \frac{\mu\lambda Ns}{\omega(\mu-\lambda Ns)}\right].$$

Find the critical value s=s* where D(s) reaches a minimum.

11. The following example illustrates the use of the conditional
    expectation given that U is distributed according to a Poisson
    density with parameter γ:

$$P_U(u) = \frac{\gamma^u\, e^{-\gamma}}{u!} \qquad\qquad : u = 0, 1, 2, \ldots,$$

and the conditional density of W given U is Binomial with
parameters u and ρ:

$$P_{W|U}(w|u) = \binom{u}{w}\rho^w(1-\rho)^{u-w} : w = 0, 1, 2, \ldots, u$$

find the expected value of W:

a.. by first working out $P_W(w)$ and then finding its expectation

b. by first finding the conditional expectation of W given U
and then eliminating the conditioning.

Solutions

1a. Given:

$$y(t) = \frac{N(t)}{S(t)}$$

it follows that

$$\frac{dy}{dt} = \frac{1}{S}\frac{dN}{dt} - \frac{N}{S^2}\frac{dS}{dt}.$$

Starting from the differential equation

$$\frac{dS}{dt} = -pS + \frac{S}{N}\frac{dN}{dt} + pS^2/mN$$

rearrange and multiply through by N/S^2:

$$\frac{1}{S}\frac{dN}{dt} - \frac{N}{S^2}\frac{dS}{dt} = pN/S - p/m.$$

Thus, using the above definitions

$$\frac{dy}{dt} = py - p/m.$$

1b. Solve the differential equation

$$\frac{dy}{dt} - py = -p/m.$$

Since $N(0) = S(0)$, $y(0) = 1$. This is the initial condition. Solve using an integrating factor

$$\frac{d}{dt}\left[ye^{-pt}\right] = -(p/m)e^{-pt}.$$

Integrate to get

$$ye^{-pt} = \frac{1}{m} e^{-pt} + C : C = \text{constant of integration.}$$

Using $y(0) = 1 \Rightarrow C = 1 - 1/m$, so

$$y(t) = \frac{1}{m} + (1 - 1/m)e^{+pt} = N/S,$$

thus

$$S = mN/[1+(m-1)e^{pt}].$$

1c. Let $D(t) = N(t) - S(t) =$ number who have had disease and survive to age t. Wish to find

$$z(t) = \frac{D(t)}{N(t)} = 1 - \frac{1}{y(t)}$$

for $t = 25$, $p = 1/8$ and $m = 8$

$$y(25) = \frac{1}{8} + (1 - \frac{1}{8})e^{25/8} = 20.04.$$

Thus

$$z(t) = 1 - \frac{1}{20.04} = .95.$$

1d. If we start by immunizing half the population in cohort, $N(0) = 2S(0) \Rightarrow y(0) = 2$. From part b, re-evaluate constant of integration $\rightarrow C = 2 - 1/m$

$$y(t) = \frac{1}{m} + (2 - 1/m)e^{pt}$$

$$y(25) = \frac{1}{8} + (2 - \frac{1}{8})e^{25/8} = 42.80$$

$$z(25) = 1 - \frac{1}{42.80} = .98.$$

1e. $y(t) = \frac{1}{m} + (1 - \frac{1}{m})e^{pt}$

$$m \rightarrow 1 \Rightarrow y(t) \rightarrow 1 \Rightarrow \frac{S(t)}{N(t)} \rightarrow 1.$$

Nobody recovers - so all alive are susceptible.

$$m \rightarrow \infty \Rightarrow y(t) \rightarrow e^{pt} \Rightarrow \frac{S(t)}{N(t)} \rightarrow e^{-pt}.$$

Everybody starts susceptible and as time passes everybody eventually contracts and recovers from smallpox.

2. To make M, ϵ and α consistent

$$(1-\epsilon)^M = (1-\alpha) \Rightarrow M \ln (1-\epsilon) = \ln (1-\alpha)$$

$$\epsilon = 1 - \exp \{\ln (1-\alpha)/M\} : M = 1000, \alpha = .001$$

$$\varepsilon = 1 \times 10^{-6}$$

$$\text{Prob}\{1 \text{ case}\} = \binom{1000}{1} \varepsilon (1-\varepsilon)^{999}$$

$$\text{Prob}\{2 \text{ cases}\} = \binom{1000}{2} \varepsilon^2 (1-\varepsilon)^{998}$$

$$\frac{\text{Prob}\{2 \text{ case}\}}{\text{Prob}\{1 \text{ case}\}} = \binom{999}{2}\varepsilon/(1-\varepsilon) \doteq .0005 = 5 \times 10^{-4}.$$

Thus the probability of 2 cases is only 5×10^{-4} as likely as of 1 case.

3. Given: $P_r = (1-\alpha)^{r-1}\alpha$

$$E\{r\} = \sum_{r=0}^{\infty} r(1-\alpha)^{r-1}\alpha = \alpha \sum_{r=0}^{\infty} r(1-\alpha)^{r-1}$$

$$= -\alpha \sum_{r=0}^{\infty} \frac{d}{d\alpha}(1-\alpha)^r = -\alpha\frac{d}{d\alpha} \sum_{r=0}^{\infty} (1-\alpha)^r$$

$$= -\alpha\frac{d}{d\alpha} \left[\frac{1}{1-(1-\alpha)}\right] = -\alpha\frac{d}{d\alpha}\left(\frac{1}{\alpha}\right) = \frac{1}{\alpha}.$$

4. Given: $\text{Prob}\{m|r\} = \binom{rV}{m}\beta^m(1-\beta)^{rV-m}$

$$E\{m|r\} = \sum_{m=0}^{rV} m\binom{rV}{m}\beta^m(1-\beta)^{rV-m}$$

but

$$m\binom{rV}{m} = \frac{m(rV)!}{m!(rV-m)!} = \frac{rV(rV-1)!}{(m-1)!(rV-m)!} = rV\binom{rV-1}{m-1}.$$

Thus

$$E\{m|r\} = rV\beta\underbrace{\sum_{m=1}^{rV} \binom{rV-1}{m-1}\beta^{m-1}(1-\beta)^{rV-m}}_{\text{1:(Sum of binomial density)}} = rV\beta.$$

5. Given: $\text{Prob}\{\text{incubation period ends}\} = \omega e^{-\omega t}$

Find: $E\{\text{length of incubation period}\}$

$$= \int_0^{\infty} \omega t e^{-\omega t}dt.$$

Integrate by parts: $u = \omega t \rightarrow du = \omega dt$

$$dv = e^{-\omega t}dt \rightarrow v = -\frac{1}{\omega}e^{-\omega t}$$

$$E\{\text{length}\} = \underbrace{-te^{-\omega t}\Big|_0^{\infty}}_{0} + \int_0^{\infty} e^{-\omega t}dt$$

$$= - \frac{1}{\omega} e^{-\omega t} \Big|_0^\infty = \frac{1}{\omega} \ .$$

6. $p_y(t+\Delta t) = p_y(t)[1-\lambda n y \Delta t - \omega y \Delta t]$

$$+ \ p_{y-1}(t)[\lambda n(y-1)\Delta t] + p_{y+1}(t)[\omega(y+1)\Delta t]$$

rearrange and let $\Delta t \to 0$

$$\frac{dp_y}{dt} = \lambda n(y-1)p_{y-1} - (\lambda n + \omega)y p_y + \omega(y+1)p_{y+1}.$$

7. $E\{Y\} = \sum\limits_{y=0}^\infty \sum\limits_{z=0}^\infty y p_{y,z}, \quad E\{Z\} = \sum\limits_{y=0}^\infty \sum\limits_{z=0}^\infty z p_{y,z}$

$$\frac{dp_{y,z}}{dt} = \lambda n(y-1)p_{y-1,z-1} - (\lambda n + \mu)y \ p_{y,z} + \mu(y+1)p_{y+1,z}.$$

a. $\dfrac{dE\{Y\}}{dt} = \sum\limits_{y=0}^\infty \sum\limits_{z=0}^\infty y \dfrac{dp_{y,z}}{dt}$

$$= \sum_{y=0}^\infty \sum_{z=0}^\infty \{\lambda n y(y-1)p_{y-1,z-1} - (\lambda n + \mu)y^2 p_{y,z}$$

$$+ \ \mu y(y+1)p_{y+1,z}\}$$

$$= \lambda n \sum_{i=0}^\infty \sum_{j=0}^\infty \underbrace{[(i+1)i - i^2]}_{i} p_{i,j} - \mu \sum_{i=0}^\infty \sum_{j=0}^\infty \underbrace{[i^2 - (i-1)i]}_{i} p_{ij}$$

$$= \lambda n E\{Y\} - \mu E\{Y\} = (n\lambda - \mu)E\{Y\}.$$

b. $\dfrac{dE\{Z\}}{dt} = \sum\limits_{y=0}^\infty \sum\limits_{z=0}^\infty z \dfrac{dp_{y,z}}{dt}$

$$= \sum_{y=0}^\infty \sum_{z=0}^\infty \{\lambda n z(y-1)p_{y-1,z-1} - (\lambda n + \mu)yz p_{y,z} + \mu z(y+1)p_{y+1,z}$$

$$= \lambda n \sum_{i=0}^\infty \sum_{j=0}^\infty \underbrace{[i(j+1) - ij]}_{i} p_{i,j} - \mu \sum_{i=0}^\infty \sum_{j=0}^\infty \underbrace{[ij - ij]}_{0} p_{i,j}$$

$$= \lambda n E\{Y\}.$$

8. $\quad I = \displaystyle\int_0^\infty \frac{(\lambda n t)^j e^{-\lambda n t}}{j!} \ \mu e^{-\mu t} dt$

$$= \frac{\mu(n\lambda)^j}{j!} \int_0^\infty t^j e^{-(n\lambda+\mu)t} dt$$

Integrate by parts: $u = t^j \longrightarrow du = jt^{j-1}dt$

$$dv = e^{-(n\lambda+\mu)t}dt \to v = \frac{-1}{(n\lambda+\mu)}e^{-(n\lambda+\mu)}$$

$$I = \frac{\mu(n\lambda)^j}{j!} \left\{ \underbrace{\frac{-t^j}{n\lambda+\mu} e^{-(n\lambda+\mu)t} \Big|_0^\infty}_{0} + \frac{j}{(n\lambda+\mu)} \int_0^\infty t^{j-1} e^{-(n\lambda+\mu)t} dt \right.$$

$$= \frac{\mu(n\lambda)^j}{(j-1)!(n\lambda+\mu)} \int_0^\infty t^{j-1} e^{-(n\lambda+\mu)t} dt$$

Repeat (j-1) more time →

$$I = \frac{\mu(n\lambda)^j}{(n\lambda+\mu)^j} \int_0^\infty e^{-(n\lambda+\mu)t} dt = \left(\frac{\mu}{n\lambda+\mu}\right)\left(\frac{n\lambda}{n\lambda+\mu}\right)^j$$

9. $E\{W_m\} = \theta\, E\{W_{m-1}\}$ and $E\{W_0\} = 0$

$E\{W_1\} = \theta\, E\{W_0\} = \theta$

$E\{W_2\} = \theta\, E\{W_1\} = \theta \cdot \theta = \theta^2$

.

.

.

$E\{W_m\} = \theta\, E\{W_{m-1}\} = \ldots = \theta^m$

10. $D(S) = \dfrac{\beta N}{\alpha} \dfrac{1-\ell+\ell/k}{365} (1-s) + \nu\left[1 + \dfrac{\mu\lambda Ns}{\omega(\mu-\lambda Ns)}\right]$

$$\frac{dD}{dt} = -\frac{\beta N}{\alpha} \frac{1-\ell+\ell/k}{365} + \left[\frac{\omega(\mu-\lambda Ns)\mu\lambda N + (\mu\lambda Ns)\omega\lambda N}{\omega^2(\mu-\lambda Ns)^2}\right] = 0$$

$$\frac{\beta N}{\alpha} \frac{1-\ell+\ell/k}{365} = \frac{\nu}{\omega} \frac{\mu^2\lambda N}{(\mu-\lambda Ns)^2}$$

Thus

$$(\mu-\lambda Ns)^2 = \frac{365\nu\alpha\mu^2\lambda}{\beta\omega(1-\ell+\ell/k)}$$

$$s = \frac{\mu}{\lambda N}\left\{1 - \sqrt{\frac{365\alpha\lambda\nu}{\omega\beta(1-\ell+\ell/k)}}\right\}$$

11a. $P_W(w) = \displaystyle\sum_{u=w}^\infty \binom{u}{w} \rho^w (1-\rho)^{u-w} \gamma^u e^{-\gamma}/u!$

$$= \frac{(\gamma\rho)^w e^{-\gamma}}{w!} \underbrace{\sum_{u=w}^\infty \frac{[\gamma(1-\rho)]^{u-w}}{(u-w)!}}_{e^{\gamma(1-\rho)}}$$

$$= \frac{(\gamma\rho)^w e^{-\gamma\rho}}{w!} \quad \text{:Poisson with parameter } \gamma\rho$$

$$E\{W\} = \sum_w wP_W(w)$$

$$= \sum_{w=1}^{\infty} \frac{(\gamma\rho)^w e^{-\gamma\rho}}{(w-1)!} = \gamma\rho$$

11b. $E\{W|U=u\} = \sum_w wP_{W|U}(w|u)$

$$= \sum_{w=0}^{u} w\binom{u}{w}\rho^w(1-\rho)^{u-w}$$

$$= \sum_{w=1}^{u} u\binom{u-1}{w-1}\rho^w(1-\rho)^{u-w} = u\rho.$$

$E\{W\} = E\{E\{W|U=u\}\}$

$$= \sum_u E\{W|U=u\}\, P_U(u)$$

$$= \sum_{u=0}^{\infty} u\rho\, \frac{\gamma^u e^{-\gamma}}{u!} = \gamma\rho.$$